THE CANCER-FIGHTING JUICE HANDBOOK

"Using Juicing for Healing and Wellness"

Peter Miller

Table Of Content

INTRODUCTION

Cancer is a devastating illness that affects millions of people around the world. While there are many conventional treatments available, many individuals are turning to alternative methods to help support their healing and improve their overall health and wellness. Juicing is one such alternative that has gained popularity for its ability to nourish the body with essential vitamins, minerals, and phytochemicals that help support healing and prevent illness.

This book, "The Cancer-Fighting Juice Handbook: Using Juicing for Healing and Wellness," is a comprehensive guide that explores the use of juicing as a tool in the fight against cancer. The book covers everything from the basic principles of juicing to the specific recipes and ingredients that have been shown to have cancer-fighting properties. It is a must-read for anyone looking to use juicing to support their healing journey and improve their overall health and wellness. Whether you are looking to prevent cancer, support recovery from conventional treatments, or simply improve your overall health and wellbeing, this book will provide you with the tools and information you need to get started. So, grab your juicer and let's get started on your journey to healthier, happier, and cancer-free life!

CHAPTER ONE
Understanding Cancer and its Causes

Cancer is a disease that affects millions of people worldwide and has been the subject of intense research and study for many years. In order to effectively combat cancer and promote healing, it is important to have a basic understanding of the disease and its causes.

This chapter will provide a comprehensive overview of the basics of cancer and its different types. The various risk factors for developing cancer will also be discussed, as well as the role that nutrition plays in both preventing and treating the disease.

The Basics of Cancer

Cancer is a group of diseases that is characterized by the uncontrolled growth and spread of abnormal cells. There are many different types of cancer, each of which can affect different parts of the body. Some common types of cancer include breast, lung, prostate, colon, and skin cancer.

Risk Factors for Developing Cancer

There are many risk factors that can increase a person's likelihood of developing cancer. Some of these risk factors include age, family history, lifestyle factors (such as smoking, alcohol consumption, and poor diet), exposure to certain chemicals and toxins, and certain medical conditions.

The Role of Nutrition in Cancer Prevention and Treatment

Nutrition plays a crucial role in both preventing and treating cancer. A diet that is high in fruits, vegetables, whole grains, and lean protein can help reduce the risk of developing cancer, while a diet that is high in processed foods, sugar, and unhealthy fats can increase the risk. In addition to this, a healthy diet can also help support the body during cancer treatment, boosting immunity, reducing inflammation, and promoting healing.

In conclusion, understanding the basics of cancer, its risk factors, and the role that nutrition plays in its prevention and treatment is an important first step in developing an effective strategy for fighting cancer. The Cancer-Fighting Juice Handbook will build on this foundation in later chapters, providing practical, actionable advice for using juicing as a tool in your journey to healing and wellness.

CHAPTER TWO
The Benefits of Juicing for Cancer

Juicing has been a popular way to improve health and wellness for many years. With the increasing interest in using natural and holistic methods to support cancer treatment, the role of juicing in cancer healing is gaining attention. In this chapter, we will explore the benefits of juicing for cancer patients and how it can support overall health and wellness.

The Benefits of Juicing for Cancer Patients

Juicing provides a concentrated source of vitamins, minerals, and antioxidants that can help boost the immune system and support the body's natural healing processes. Fresh juice is also an excellent source of enzymes, which are important for digestion and overall health. In particular, the high content of antioxidants in fresh juice can help protect cells from damage, which is particularly important for cancer patients who are undergoing treatments that can damage healthy cells.

How Juicing Can Improve Overall Health and Support Cancer Treatment

Juicing can help improve overall health by providing the body with the nutrients it needs to function optimally. This can help reduce the side effects of cancer treatments and support the body's natural healing processes. For example, fresh juice can help alleviate fatigue, improve energy levels, and boost the immune system, which can all help improve the overall quality of life for cancer patients.

The Science Behind the Healing Power of Fresh Juice

Studies have shown that the nutrients in fresh juice can have a positive impact on various aspects of health, including cancer. For example, studies have found that the antioxidants in fresh juice can help protect cells from damage, while the high content of vitamins and minerals can help support the immune system and overall health.

In conclusion, the benefits of juicing for cancer patients are clear. By providing a concentrated source of vitamins, minerals, and antioxidants, fresh juice can support the body's natural healing processes and help improve overall health and wellness.

CHAPTER THREE
Choosing the Right Juices for Cancer Healing

When it comes to juicing for cancer healing, choosing the right ingredients can make all the difference. In this chapter, we'll explore the importance of selecting nutrient-dense ingredients that are specifically targeted towards cancer support.

There are a number of different types of cancer, and each one requires a slightly different approach to treatment. This means that there are specific ingredients that are ideal for different types of cancer. For example, ingredients that are high in antioxidants are great for fighting free radicals, which can cause damage to cells and contribute to the development of cancer.

Here are some common ingredients and recipes to support specific types of cancer:

1. Antioxidant-rich juices for all types of cancer Ingredients:

- 1 large beet
- 2 large carrots
- 2 large apples
- 1 large handful of spinach
- 1 inch of fresh ginger

Instructions:

1. Wash all produce thoroughly and chop into pieces that will fit through your juicer's feed chute.

2. Run all ingredients through your juicer and mix the resulting juice together.

3. Drink immediately for best results.

4. Juices to support liver function and fight liver cancer Ingredients:

- 1 large beet
- 2 large carrots
- 2 large apples
- 1 large handful of spinach
- 1 inch of fresh ginger

- 1 large lemon, peeled

Instructions:

1. Wash all produce thoroughly and chop into pieces that will fit through your juicer's feed chute.

2. Run all ingredients through your juicer and mix the resulting juice together.

3. Drink immediately for best results.

4. Juices to support lung health and fight lung cancer Ingredients:

- 2 large carrots

- 1 large apple

- 2 large handfuls of kale

- 1 large handful of parsley

- 1 inch of fresh ginger

- 1 lemon, peeled

Instructions:

1. Wash all produce thoroughly and chop into pieces that will fit through your juicer's feed chute.

2. Run all ingredients through your juicer and mix the resulting juice together.

3. Drink immediately for best results.

When it comes to creating a delicious, nutrient-dense juice, it's important to balance flavors and ingredients. This means that you'll want to choose ingredients that complement each other, both in terms of taste and health benefits. For example, adding ginger to your juice can help to improve digestion and enhance the flavor, while adding lemon can add a tart and refreshing element to the drink.

With these recipes and tips in mind, you're well on your way to creating delicious, cancer-fighting juices that can help to improve your overall health and support your healing journey.

CHAPTER FOUR
Incorporating Juicing into Your Cancer Treatment Plan

Focusing on the importance of working with your healthcare team to integrate juicing into your cancer treatment plan. This chapter provides a comprehensive guide to understanding the benefits and limitations of juicing for cancer, as well as tips for fitting juicing into your daily routine.

One of the first steps in incorporating juicing into your cancer treatment plan is to talk to your healthcare team about your goals and how juicing can fit into your overall treatment strategy. It's important to understand that while juicing can provide many health benefits, it is not a cure for cancer and should be used in conjunction with other treatments, such as chemotherapy, radiation, or surgery.

Once you've discussed your goals and treatment plan with your healthcare team, you can start to think about how to fit juicing into your daily routine. This may involve planning ahead and setting aside time each day for juicing, as well as considering the equipment and ingredients you'll need. Some people prefer to juice at home, while others find it more convenient to purchase pre-made juices or attend a juice bar.

When it comes to choosing the right juices for cancer healing, it's important to focus on nutrient-dense ingredients that have been shown to have anti-cancer properties. Some of the best ingredients for cancer-fighting juices include:

- Leafy greens such as spinach, kale, and chard, which are high in vitamins, minerals, and antioxidants.

- Berries such as blueberries, raspberries, and blackberries, which are high in antioxidants and phytochemicals.

- Cruciferous vegetables such as broccoli, cauliflower, and cabbage, which contain anti-cancer compounds such as sulforaphane and indole-3-carbinol.

- Spices such as turmeric, ginger, and garlic, which have anti-inflammatory and antioxidant properties.

When juicing, it's also important to balance flavors and ingredients to create tasty, healing juices that are easy to drink. Some of the most popular and delicious juice recipes for cancer healing include:

- Green Machine: This juice combines spinach, kale, cucumber, apple, lemon, and ginger for a nutrient-dense and refreshing drink.

- Berry Blast: This juice blends blueberries, raspberries, blackberries, and lemon for a sweet and tangy drink that's high in antioxidants.

- Cruciferous Cocktail: This juice combines broccoli, cauliflower, cabbage, apple, and ginger for a veggie-packed drink that's full of anti-cancer compounds.

- Spice it Up: This juice combines turmeric, ginger, garlic, lemon, and honey for a spicy and healing drink that's great for reducing inflammation and boosting immunity.

Incorporating juicing into your cancer treatment plan can be a powerful tool for supporting your overall health and wellness. By focusing on nutrient-dense ingredients, balancing flavors and ingredients, and working with your healthcare team, you can create a juicing routine that's tailored to your specific needs and goals.

CHAPTER FIVE
Supporting Your Body and Mind with Juicing

Cancer treatment can be an intense and challenging experience, both physically and emotionally. The stress and anxiety that often accompany a cancer diagnosis can have a significant impact on the body's ability to heal. However, incorporating healthy habits, such as juicing, can help to support both the body and mind during this time.

The role of juicing in promoting relaxation and stress relief

Juicing can play a critical role in promoting relaxation and stress relief, as certain ingredients can help to reduce anxiety and promote feelings of calmness. For example, ingredients such as chamomile, lavender, and passionflower have been shown to have calming effects on the mind and body. Additionally, the high concentration of vitamins and nutrients in fresh juice can help to boost the immune system, which can in turn help to reduce stress and support overall health.

Supporting the body's natural healing processes with juicing

Incorporating juicing into your cancer treatment plan can also help to support the body's natural healing processes. The high concentration of vitamins, minerals, and antioxidants in fresh juice can help to boost the immune system, reduce inflammation, and protect against oxidative stress. This can be particularly important for cancer patients, who often have weakened immune systems due to the treatments they are undergoing.

By incorporating a variety of nutrient-dense ingredients into your juicing routine, you can support your body's natural healing processes and improve your overall health and well-being during your cancer journey. Whether you are seeking to reduce stress, boost your immune system, or simply improve your overall health, juicing can be a powerful tool for supporting your body and mind during this time.

CHAPTER SIX
Staying Motivated and Making Juicing a Lifestyle

Juicing can be a powerful tool in the journey of cancer healing and wellness, but it can also be challenging to maintain consistency and motivation. In this chapter, we will explore strategies for staying motivated and making juicing a lifestyle.

Overcoming challenges and staying motivated in your juicing journey

Making a commitment to juicing for cancer healing can be a big step, and it can be easy to lose motivation along the way. To overcome these challenges, it's important to set realistic goals and understand the benefits of juicing. Keeping a journal of your progress and tracking the positive changes in your body and mind can also help you stay motivated. You can also set reminders or schedule juicing sessions in advance to make sure it becomes a regular part of your routine.

Building a supportive community for cancer healing

Having a support system can be a crucial factor in staying motivated and reaching your juicing goals. Reach out to family and friends or consider joining a support group for individuals who are also on a cancer healing journey. You can also connect with others who have undergone similar experiences on online forums or social media platforms. Sharing your progress, recipes, and challenges with others can help keep you accountable and inspired.

Integrating juicing into a balanced and healthy lifestyle

Juicing can be a great addition to a healthy lifestyle, but it should not be the only approach to cancer healing. Incorporating regular exercise, getting enough sleep, and eating a well-balanced diet are also important components of a healthy lifestyle. Additionally, it's important to avoid harmful habits, such as smoking and excessive alcohol consumption, which can have a negative impact on cancer healing. By incorporating juicing into a balanced and healthy lifestyle, you can support your body's natural healing processes and optimize your overall health.

In conclusion, staying motivated and making juicing a lifestyle is an important aspect of cancer healing. By setting realistic goals, building a supportive community, and integrating juicing into a balanced and healthy lifestyle, you can reap the benefits of juicing for cancer healing and wellness.

CHAPTER SEVEN
Conclusion and Final Thoughts

In this book, we've explored the power of juicing in the fight against cancer. From understanding the basics of cancer and its causes, to exploring the benefits of juicing for cancer patients, and learning how to incorporate juicing into your cancer treatment plan, we've covered a lot of ground.

At the heart of the matter is the fact that nutrition plays a critical role in cancer healing and prevention. Fresh, nutrient-dense juices can provide the body with the nourishment it needs to support the healing process and improve overall health. Incorporating juicing into your cancer treatment plan can help to boost your immune system, improve your mental and emotional well-being, and support your body's natural healing processes.

One of the key challenges in any cancer healing journey is staying motivated and committed to a healthy lifestyle. This is where building a supportive community, finding inspiration and encouragement, and making juicing a lifelong habit can make a big difference.

In conclusion, we hope that this book has been a valuable resource for you on your journey to cancer healing and wellness. Whether you are a cancer patient, a caregiver, or someone looking to improve your overall health and prevent cancer, we wish you continued success and growth on your journey. Remember to listen to your body, be kind to yourself, and never give up. The power of juicing is in your hands.